Effective Ways to Prevent Unplanned Pregnancy Naturally

Sam Skinner

Acknowledgement

I would like to express my sincere gratitude to all those who have contributed to this project. Your dedication, support, and expertise have been invaluable in bringing our vision to fruition. I am truly thankful for the collaborative spirit and unwavering commitment demonstrated by each member of the team. Together, we have achieved remarkable results that will have a lasting impact. Thank you for your hard work and dedication.

Dedication

To my dearest father, and Wife.

Your unwavering support and boundless love have been the cornerstone of my journey. Through your guidance and encouragement, I've discovered strength and resilience beyond measure. Each of you has played an integral role in shaping who I am today, and for that, I am forever grateful.

To my cherished wife,

You are the heartbeat of our family, the pillar of strength in times of need, and the beacon of light that guides me through darkness. Your unwavering love, patience, and understanding have been my greatest blessings. With you by my side, I am whole, and every challenge becomes conquerable. I am forever grateful for your love and devotion.

Sadiq Inuwa

Table of Contents

Chapter One

Exploring Herbal Remedies and Supplements

1. **Introduction**

In today's environment, people seek natural solutions for a variety of issues, including contraception. While there are several contraceptive methods available, some people wish to forgo synthetic hormones or devices. This post will look at natural ways to avoid getting pregnant after sex.

Understanding reproductive: Before getting into natural contraceptive options, it's important to understand reproductive cycles. Women are most fertile during ovulation, which usually happens in the middle of their menstrual cycle. Recognizing indications of ovulation, such as changes in cervical mucus or basal body temperature, might help you determine fertile days.

The timing or calendar approach involves charting menstrual cycles to determine fertile and infertile days. Individuals can naturally minimize their risk of conception by refraining from having intercourse during fertile periods. However, this strategy necessitates constancy and accuracy in monitoring menstrual cycles.

Herbal Remedies: Certain herbs and plants are thought to contain contraceptive qualities. For example, Queen Anne's Lace (Daucus carota) seeds have long been used as a natural contraceptive. However, the efficacy and safety of herbal contraception therapies have not been thoroughly examined and may differ between individuals.

nursing: Exclusive nursing, also known as lactational amenorrhea, might suppress ovulation and delay the resumption of menstruation in certain women. This natural method of contraception, also known as the lactational amenorrhea method (LAM), is most successful when certain conditions are satisfied, such as exclusive nursing and the absence of menstruation.

Chapter Two

2. Understanding Natural Methods of Pregnancy Prevention

Exploring natural techniques is the greatest and least harmful way to avoid pregnancy. Let's define some words using natural methods.

Fertility awareness method (FAM)

The Fertility Awareness Method (FAM) is a natural family planning strategy that includes recording numerous indications and symptoms during a woman's menstrual cycle to identify fertile and infertile periods. These symptoms may include changes in cervical mucus consistency, basal body temperature, and cervical posture. FAM may be used to obtain or prevent pregnancy by determining when ovulation occurs and fertility is greatest. It requires regular monitoring and comprehension of one's menstrual cycle.

Basal body temperature (BBT) tracking

Basal body temperature (BBT) monitoring is a fertility awareness technique that measures a woman's body temperature at rest, usually first thing in the morning before engaging in any physical activity. BBT often rises significantly after ovulation owing to the release of progesterone, a hormone that raises metabolic rate. Individuals who record daily temperatures throughout the menstrual cycle may find trends and determine when ovulation occurs, allowing them to anticipate fertile and infertile periods for pregnancy prevention or conception.

Cervical mucus observation
Cervical mucus observation is a fertility awareness technique that tracks changes in the quality and amount of cervical mucus during a woman's menstrual cycle. The cervix generates many forms of mucus in

response to hormonal fluctuations. As ovulation approaches, estrogen levels increase, leading cervical mucus to become clearer, stretchier, and more copious, much like raw egg whites. This fertile-type mucus promotes sperm survival and transit, signifying the most fertile time for conception. Following ovulation, progesterone dominance leads the mucus to thicken and become less elastic, forming a natural barrier to sperm. Observing these variations allows people to determine fertile and infertile periods for pregnancy avoidance or conception.

Calendar-Based and Fertility Awareness-Based Methods
Calendar-based methods
Calendar-based approaches, such as the Rhythm Method, follow a woman's menstrual cycle to determine when she is most likely to get pregnant and are the oldest kind of natural family planning.

Fertility Awareness-Based Methods (FABMs) usually monitor changes in one or more fertility indicators related with ovulation: basal body temperature, cervical mucus, hormone production, and cervical position, however they may also involve calendar monitoring. The basal body temperature (BBT) approach needs a woman to measure her temperature every morning as soon as she wakes up, before getting out of bed, while the cervical mucus monitoring method requires her to document changes in vaginal discharge every day. Sympto-thermal approaches follow numerous signals, most often the BBT and cervical mucus monitoring methods, and are thought to be more successful than utilizing just one of them. Other techniques may measure hormone levels in the urine as well as changes in cervix position.

Breastfeeding may also be used as a form of contraception for postpartum women. Lactation amenorrhea is a short period of infertility that occurs soon after a baby is born, during which the hormones that create breast milk block ovulation. To be successful with this type of contraception, a mother must solely and regularly nurse her infant for up to 6 months, or until her period returns. This strategy does not work for ladies who use a breast pump or formula.

Table 1: Natural Family Planning and Fertility Awareness Methods

Types	protocol	Method.	Days to avoid unprotected sex
Tracking Days of	Calendar Rhythm Method	Track cycle lengths to calculate	Avoid unprotected sex during

| Menstrual Cycle | Standard Days Method (SDM) | fertile windows.

Avoid unprotected sex on days 8-19 of the cycle. | the fertile window. |
| Cervical Mucus Monitoring (CMM) | Billings Ovulation Method

Creighton Model Fertilitycare System (CrMS)

Two-Day Method (TDM) | Monitor characteristics of cervical mucus (vaginal discharge) daily Monitor cervical mucus daily; use a more detailed classification system

Check cervical mucus secretions at least twice a day. | Any day with menstruation or secretion; Alternate sexual intercourse during "infertile days" If cervical secretions are present "today" or "yesterday" |

Temperature	Basal Body Temperature Method (BBT)	Take and chart temperature every morning before getting out of bed to identify a postovulatory increase in temperature.	Avoid sex from the start of menstruation until three days after seeing the temperature rise.
Multiple Indicators	Sympto-Thermal Method (STM) Sympto-hormonal Method (Marquette Model, Persona)	Combines BBT and CMM Combines the CMM with a fertility monitor that measures hormones present in the urine.	During the fertile window identified by the various markers.
Postpartum	Lactation Amenorrhea Method	Exclusively breastfeed baby up to 6 months	None until the period returns.

	(LAM)	postpartum (or until period returns)	

Use and Efficacy

The use of natural family planning techniques in the United States is low. In 2014, an estimated 2% of sexually active women aged 15-44 utilized a natural family planning strategy.2 Women may choose these procedures because they are hormone-free, inexpensive, or for religious or personal reasons. The average efficiency of NFP techniques in preventing pregnancy is determined by the accuracy of the method used, the woman's ability to accurately read biological signals of fertility, and the couple's ability to avoid unprotected sex within the fertile window (Table 2). Clinical investigations indicate that NFP approaches fail relatively seldom when used correctly.

However, perfect utilization is difficult to attain. There is plenty of possibility for human mistake, and even a single miscalculation might result in an unplanned pregnancy. Furthermore, several clinical studies evaluating the effectiveness of these approaches have been questioned for reporting low failure rates owing to selection bias and non-representative populations.3 A recent systematic review discovered that there are few research testing the usefulness of fertility awareness-based approaches, and those that do exist are of moderate to poor quality. Overall, NFP approaches have a failure rate of up to 25 pregnancies per 100 women each year.4 Lactation amenorrhea, on the other hand, is particularly successful for around 6 months after childbirth, provided that an Omani exclusively breastfeeds her newborn.

Ovulation predictor kits (OPKs)

Ovulation Predictor Kits (OPKs) are home testing kits that help people who are attempting to conceive or prevent pregnancy forecast when they will ovulate. These assays detect the spike in luteinizing hormone (LH) levels in urine, which usually occurs 24-48 hours before ovulation. OPKs recognize this LH surge, which helps pinpoint the most fertile window during a woman's menstrual cycle, allowing people to schedule intercourse for conception or use contraception to prevent pregnancy. OPKs are simple to use and provide a handy way to monitor ovulation at home.

Withdrawal method (pull-out method)

The withdrawal method, also known as the pull-out method, is a contraceptive procedure in which the male partner removes his penis from the vagina before ejaculating during sexual intercourse. The purpose is to prevent sperm from entering the vagina and reaching the egg, therefore lowering the chance of pregnancy. However, this procedure is not very successful since sperm might be present in pre-ejaculatory fluid and correct timing of withdrawal is difficult. As a result, it is regarded as one of the least dependable means of contraception and provides no protection against sexually transmitted diseases (STIs).

Abstinence

Abstinence is the choice to abstain from participating in sexual activity, which usually includes vaginal, oral, or anal intercourse. It is a kind of contraception and STI prevention strategy that entails refraining from any sexual contact with a partner. Abstinence is thought to be 100% effective in avoiding pregnancy and STIs when maintained continuously. It is often offered as a safe and dependable choice for those who are not ready for or do not want to participate in sexual activity.

The lactational amenorrhea method (LAM)

The Lactational Amenorrhea Method (LAM) is a natural type of birth control utilized by nursing moms throughout the postpartum period. It is based on the temporary infertility that nursing might cause owing to hormonal changes. LAM is founded on three criteria: exclusive breastfeeding (feeding the baby just breast milk, no other liquids or solids), amenorrhea (lack of menstrual periods), and the infant's age less than six months. When these parameters are satisfied, LAM may be a very effective form of contraception. However, when any of these conditions change, the efficacy of LAM declines, and alternative contraceptive methods may be required to avoid pregnancy.

Chapter three

3 **Herbal Remedies for Pregnancy Prevention**

Herbal treatments have been used for ages as a form of contraception and pregnancy prevention. These therapies often include the use of different plants, herbs, and natural compounds said to have contraceptive effects. Some herbal cures for pregnancy prevention have been handed down through generations and are based on traditional knowledge, while others have acquired popularity via contemporary study and testing.

Herbal therapies for pregnancy prevention may act via a variety of ways, including regulating hormone levels, influencing sperm motility and viability, and producing an unfavorable environment for fertilization or implantation. However, it is important to remember that the efficiency and safety of herbal contraception may vary greatly, and not all therapies are scientifically proven.

Common herbal medicines for pregnancy prevention include neem, wild yam, Queen Anne's lace, and pennyroyal. These plants are thought to have contraceptive properties and are often used in the form of teas, tinctures, and supplements. Furthermore, some herbal combinations or formulations may be advised due to their synergistic benefits in preventing pregnancy.

While herbal therapies for pregnancy prevention provide a natural alternative to conventional contraceptives, they should be used with care. To ensure safety, effectiveness, and correct use, consult with a healthcare physician or herbalist who specializes in reproductive health. Individuals should also be aware of possible negative effects, drug interactions, and the significance of utilizing backup contraception while using herbal medicines alone.

Overall, herbal therapies for pregnancy prevention may be a realistic choice for those looking for natural contraceptives. However, comprehensive research, intelligent decision-making, and expert supervision are required to enhance their efficacy and reduce possible hazards.

3.2 Hormone Balancing Herbs

Hormone-balancing herbs are natural compounds obtained from plants and herbs that are thought to help control hormone levels in the body. These herbs are often used to treat hormonal imbalances that may lead to a variety of health problems, such as menstruation irregularities, fertility concerns, menopausal symptoms, and hormonal acne.

Some common hormone-balancing herbs include:

1. Vitex (Chaste tree berry): Helps with hormonal balance, especially in situations of irregular menstruation, premenstrual syndrome (PMS), and infertility.
2. Dong Quai, sometimes known as "female ginseng," is a traditional Chinese medicine herb used to regulate menstrual cycles, reduce menstrual cramps, and promote general reproductive health.
3. Maca root: Maca root is believed to help regulate hormones and promote fertility, as well as to boost vitality and adaptability.
4. Black cohosh is used to help with menopausal symptoms including hot flashes, night sweats, and mood swings by balancing hormone levels.

5. Red clover contains phytoestrogens, which may help relieve menopausal symptoms and maintain hormonal balance in women.

6. Ashwagandha is an adaptogenic plant that helps the body adapt to stress and may promote hormone balance by lowering cortisol levels.

7. Rhodiola: Rhodiola is another adaptogenic herb that helps the body adapt to stress. It may indirectly promote hormone balance by lowering stress levels.

8. Wild yam contains diosgenin, a chemical thought to have hormone-balancing properties and promote menstrual regularity.

9. Tribulus is used to improve reproductive health and hormone balance, especially in males, by raising testosterone levels.

10. Licorice root: Promotes adrenal gland function and may help regulate hormone levels, notably cortisol.

It is crucial to remember that, although hormone-balancing herbs are extensively used and generally regarded safe, they may not be appropriate for everyone. Individuals with hormone-related problems or who are on drugs should check with a healthcare provider before introducing these herbs into their routine. Furthermore, herbal medicines should be taken carefully and in moderation, since they may cause negative effects or interactions with drugs.

.

3.3. Herbs with Antifertility Properties
1. Neem (Azadirachta indica) has been utilized as a contraceptive in many cultures owing to its spermicidal and anti-implantation properties.

2. Queen Anne's lace (Daucus carota): Also known as wild carrot, Queen Anne's lace is said to have contraceptive effects, however its effectiveness has not been proven.

3. Papaya seeds contain enzymes that may reduce sperm motility and viability, thus acting as a contraceptive.

4. Smartweed (Polygonum hydropiper) has long been used as a contraceptive owing to its ability to prevent implantation.

5. Wild yam (Dioscorea villosa) includes diosgenin, a chemical that is thought to have contraceptive properties by changing hormone levels and interfering with ovulation.

6. Blue cohosh (Caulophyllum thalictroides) has long been used to

induce menstruation and may have antifertility properties, while its safety and efficiency are unknown.

7. Pennyroyal (Mentha pulegium) oil has long been used as a contraceptive, however it is poisonous and should be taken with great care.

8. Rue (Ruta graveolens): Rue has historically been used as a contraceptive and abortifacient, however it is hazardous and should be handled with care.

9.

Supplements for Pregnancy Prevention

While certain supplements may have qualities that might help with pregnancy prevention, it is important to emphasize that they are not dependable as independent contraception techniques. Always get advice from a healthcare professional before using contraception. The following supplements have been proposed to have possible impacts on fertility or hormone balance, however their efficacy as contraceptives may vary:

1. Vitamin C: According to some research, excessive amounts of vitamin C may inhibit progesterone production, thereby disrupting the menstrual cycle and ovulation. However, further study is required to validate its contraceptive effectiveness.

2. Vitamin E is thought to have antioxidant qualities that may benefit reproductive health, although its involvement in pregnancy prevention is not fully understood.

3. Zinc has a critical function in reproductive health and hormone balance. While zinc deficiency may

reduce fertility, there is no evidence of its direct contraceptive effects.

4. Omega-3 fatty acids: Omega-3 fatty acids, found in fish oil and some plant sources, are beneficial to general health, including reproductive function. Some studies show that omega-3 supplementation may aid fertility, although its function in pregnancy prevention is not fully understood.

5. Evening primrose oil includes gamma-linolenic acid (GLA), which is thought to promote hormonal balance. Some women take it to treat premenstrual syndrome (PMS) or irregular menstrual cycles, although its contraceptive efficacy is unknown.

6. Vitex (Chaste tree berry) is a popular plant that is said to help with

hormonal balance and menstrual cycle regulation. While some women take it to improve fertility or relieve PMS symptoms, its function in pregnancy prevention is unclear.

7. Dong Quai is a plant that has long been used in Chinese medicine to improve women's health and control menstrual cycles. Some women take it to increase their fertility, although its contraceptive effects are not well proven.

Supplements should not be used as main contraceptive techniques. While certain supplements may affect fertility or hormone balance, they are not a replacement for effective contraception, such as hormonal contraceptives, barrier techniques, or intrauterine devices (IUDs). Consult a healthcare provider for tailored advice on contraception and reproductive health.

Chapter Four

4.1. **Vitamins and Minerals**

Vitamins and minerals are crucial for general health and may indirectly affect fertility and reproductive health. While they are not independent contraceptives, maintaining proper amounts of key vitamins and minerals is critical for reproductive health. The following vitamins and minerals are especially crucial for reproductive health:

1. Folic acid (vitamin B9) is essential for fetal development and may help avoid neural tube abnormalities in growing babies. It is suggested that women of reproductive age take enough folic acid before and throughout pregnancy.

2. Iron is required for the formation of healthy red blood cells as well as the prevention of anemia, which may have an impact on fertility and pregnancy outcomes. Women with iron deficiency may have irregular menstrual periods or problems conceiving.

3. Vitamin D: Vitamin D helps regulate hormones and may affect fertility. Some studies imply that vitamin D insufficiency is linked to infertility, but further study is required to fully understand the association.

4. Zinc is required for reproductive health in both men and women. It helps regulate hormones, produce sperm, and mature eggs. Zinc insufficiency may reduce fertility in both sexes.

5. Omega-3 fatty acids, such as EPA and DHA, are beneficial to general health

and may aid with conception by lowering inflammation and promoting hormone balance. Flaxseeds, walnuts, and fatty salmon are all good sources.

6. Vitamin E, an antioxidant, may protect reproductive cells from free radical damage. Some studies indicate that vitamin E administration may increase sperm quality and fertility in males.

7. Vitamin C: Vitamin C is an antioxidant that may preserve sperm from oxidative damage and increase their quality. Some research suggests that vitamin C intake may improve sperm motility and prevent sperm DNA damage.

8. Selenium: Selenium is a trace mineral that affects sperm production and quality. Adequate selenium levels may promote male fertility.

9. Magnesium is involved in many metabolic activities in the body, such as hormone control and muscle function. It may indirectly affect fertility by improving general health and hormone balance.

10. B vitamins, such as B6, B12, and riboflavin (B2), play vital roles in energy metabolism and hormone control. Adequate B vitamin consumption is critical for general health and may indirectly promote fertility.

While maintaining appropriate amounts of vitamins and minerals is vital for reproductive health, they should be obtained from a well-balanced diet rather than supplements. A nutritious diet high in fruits, vegetables, whole grains, lean meats, and healthy fats may provide the nutrients required for reproductive health.

Individuals with particular vitamin shortages or health issues may benefit from supplementing when advised by a healthcare expert.

4.2 Combining Herbal Remedies and Supplements for Enhanced Effectiveness

Combining herbal treatments and supplements for increased success in fertility awareness techniques may be accomplished with careful thought and advice from a healthcare practitioner. Here are some things to bear in mind:

1. Consultation: Before mixing herbal treatments and supplements, speak with a healthcare physician or a competent herbalist to determine your specific health requirements, hormone imbalances, and possible interactions with drugs or pre-existing health concerns.

2. Personalized approach: Fertility awareness is very personalized, so what works for one person may not work for another. Collaborate with your healthcare physician to create a tailored plan that takes into consideration your reproductive goals, health state, and preferences.

3. Some herbal medicines and supplements may have complimentary effects when used together, thereby increasing their total efficacy. For example, combining herbal medicines known to assist hormone balance with nutrient-dense supplements may give overall reproductive health support.

4. Safety considerations: While herbal medicines and supplements are typically regarded as safe when taken correctly, they may nevertheless cause side effects, interactions, or unpleasant reactions. When mixing

different drugs, exercise caution and adhere to the appropriate doses and instructions supplied by your healthcare professional.

5. Monitoring and Adjustments: Keep note of how your body reacts to the combination of herbal treatments and vitamins. Keep track of changes in your menstrual cycle, fertility symptoms, and general health. If you encounter any side effects, or if your symptoms continue or worsen, see your doctor about making changes to your treatment plan.

6. Lifestyle factors: In addition to herbal treatments and supplements, food, exercise, stress management, and sleep all have a substantial influence on fertility and reproductive health. Incorporate healthy lifestyle behaviors to supplement your fertility awareness efforts and improve your general well-being.

7. Combining herbal treatments and supplements in a holistic and educated approach has the ability to improve fertility awareness practices and contribute to overall reproductive health. However, you must continue cautiously, seek expert advice, and emphasize safety and efficacy in your reproductive journey.

Conclusion:
While natural contraception techniques provide alternatives to standard contraceptives, they may be less trustworthy or successful in avoiding pregnancy. It is important to thoroughly consider the dangers and advantages of each approach before consulting with healthcare specialists for specific advice. Furthermore, combining natural techniques with barrier or fertility awareness approaches may improve contraceptive efficacy. Ultimately, making educated choices and prioritizing reproductive health are critical when navigating contraceptive alternatives.